Friend Grief and AIDS:

THIRTY YEARS OF BURYING OUR FRIENDS

VICTORIA NOE

Copyright © 2013 by Victoria Noe

Cover design: Rebecca Swift

All rights reserved. This book or any portion thereof may not be reproduced or used in any manner whatsoever without the express written permission of the publisher except for the use of brief quotations in a book review.

This book is not intended as a substitute for therapeutic or medical advice. The reader should regularly consult a medical professional in matters relating to his/her health and particularly with respect to any symptoms that may require diagnosis or medical attention.

Printed in the United States of America

First edition, 2013
Second edition, 2017

ISBNs: print – 978-0-9884632-2-6
.epub – 978-0-9884632-3-3
.mobi – 978-0-9884632-5-7

King Company Publishing – Chicago, IL 60618

www.VictoriaNoe.com

Table of Contents

Introduction: The Face of AIDS 1

In the Beginning, Friends Learned a New Alphabet 7

Why Friends Mattered – And Still Do 9

Silence=Death – How ACT UP Changed Everything 17

The Quilt and Grieving 25

Guilt/Sainthood by Association 33

The Other Kind of Guilt 35

The Glamor Quotient 39

No Big Deal Anymore, Right? 45

How We Remember Them 49

On World AIDS Day, 2016, the face of AIDS looked like this: 53

References: 55

Acknowledgements: 57

Other books by Victoria Noe: 59

About the Author 60

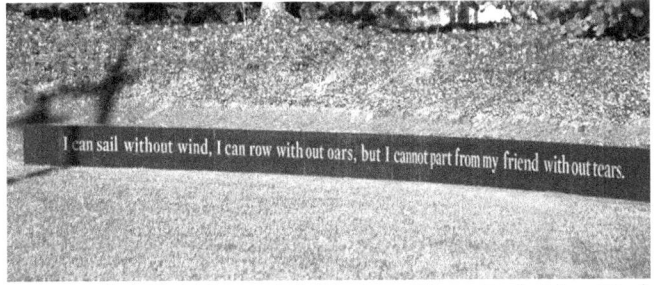

New York AIDS Memorial, Hudson River Park, New York

AIDS@30: A Time Capsule. Copyright © 2011 by Bill Hayes. By permission of *The New York Review of Books* blog, *NYRblog* (www.nyrbooks.com/blogs/nyrblog).

AIDS@30 series. Copyright ©2011. By permission of Windy City Media Group.

Love is the Cure: On Life, Loss and the End of AIDS by Elton John. Copyright © 2012 by The Elton John Foundation. By permission of Little, Brown and Company. All rights reserved.

Love is the Cure: On Life, Loss and the End of AIDS by Elton John. Copyright © 2012. Reproduced by permission of Hodder & Stoughton, Limited.

Moving Politics: Emotion and ACT UP's Fight Against AIDS. Copyright ©2009 by Deborah Gould. By permission of University of Chicago Press.

Out of My Second Closet: Memoir of an AIDS Survivor. Copyright © 2012 by Dwayne Carl. By permission of Dwayne Carl.

Introduction: The Face of AIDS

"I hope you'll still support us when the people who live at our houses don't just look like your friends."

I don't know what possessed me to say it. It was 1990 and I was the development director at Chicago House, a residential and support program for men and women living with HIV/AIDS. I'd been invited to make a presentation to a group of volunteers from DIFFA (Design Industry Foundation for AIDS), a big supporter of the cause.

I knew the face of AIDS was changing, from mostly white, gay men to every ethnic group, IV-drug users, prostitutes, women and children. Because of the large number of gay men involved in design, DIFFA was created early on in the fight against AIDS, and I appreciated their support. When I finished talking, I hoped no one had actually heard that comment.

But afterwards, an executive from DIFFA approached me.

"Thank you for saying that," he said. "It's important."

Acquired Immune Deficiency Syndrome (formerly known as GRID, ARC and Gay Cancer) is an equal-opportunity virus.

It doesn't care if you're male or female, young or old, or not yet born. It doesn't care if you're gay, straight, bisexual or transgender. It doesn't care if you're black, white, Asian, Latino or any combination. It doesn't care about your economic status, political persuasion, sports obsession, musical taste or educational level. It doesn't care if you are religious or agnostic or atheist. All it cares about is that you are human and available.

A scientist might say there's beauty in that lack of discrimination.

The photographs that were burned into our minds from the early days of the epidemic are the ones that remain with us thirty years later: a man, probably white, with an emaciated body, haunting eyes, wispy hair, dark spots on his skin. They were often compared to photos of prisoners liberated from World War II concentration camps.

I used to think of it as 'the look'. I knew when I saw someone fitting that description that his time was limited. You didn't have to know what they looked like before, when they were healthy, or seemed to be. It was the face of AIDS.

It was a national shock to the system when Rock Hudson's publicist revealed his client's AIDS diagnosis in 1985. For many people, the photos of the once-handsome movie star were their first glimpse at the physical destruction the virus could wreak.

INTRODUCTION: THE FACE OF AIDS

The problem, as we soon learned, was that the fear and hatred weren't directed only towards white, gay men. It's difficult now to understand the level of hysteria in those early days, even given the lack of scientific evidence:

Also in 1985, the Kokomo, Indiana school board banned Ryan White, a seventh grader who had contracted AIDS due to a blood transfusion, from attending classes. His family sued, and the following year he was allowed to return, with conditions: no gym class, separate bathroom, separate water fountain, plastic utensils in the cafeteria. Over two dozen children were removed from the school by their parents, who set up an alternative school for them.

But that was only part of it. Ryan's paper route customers cancelled their subscriptions. The tires on his mother's car were slashed, and someone shot a bullet into their home. Death threats – directed at the family, their friends, even a local reporter who told their story – were common.

Perhaps the saddest part of the way he was treated was that even their church abandoned him. Ryan, his mother and sister were forced to sit in either the first pew or the last, shunned by their fellow parishioners who refused to extend a handshake of peace on Easter.

He and his family endured all of this abuse and much more with grace and dignity, and a firm resolve to educate the world about this terrible disease.

Ryan was, in the parlance of the day, an "innocent victim" of AIDS. Babies born to mothers who'd been infected by their partners or through IV-drug use were also deemed innocent. Politicians and religious leaders generally drew a line as far as guilt, but failed to treat them with any more humanity.

The best and fastest way to stop the spread of AIDS in IV-drug users is by needle exchanges. Reusing needles leads to soaring infection rates of not just AIDS, but hepatitis and other diseases. Politicians across the country, at all levels of government, can't understand that needle exchanges are a positive step. All they see is a policy that encourages drug use.

Early opposition to needle exchange programs came from the African-American community. IV-drug users shared needles in 'shooting galleries' in their neighborhoods. But many strongly believed that exchanging used syringes for clean ones, and encouraging addicts to not re-use or share them, was tantamount to glorifying drug use.

There are about 200 needle exchange programs in the US, in 34 states. In 2009, President Obama signed a law to reinstate federal funding for needle exchange programs. Congress banned it again, despite the fact that these programs can reduce the rate of infection by 80%, according to the American Foundation for AIDS Research (amfAR).

Condoms were one of the first discoveries for effectively preventing transmission. But the Catholic Church could not distinguish between using condoms to prevent AIDS and using condoms to prevent pregnancy.

In 1990, Pope John Paul II insisted fidelity and abstinence were the only true ways to fight AIDS. Five years later, the Pontifical Council for the Family insisted that the whole concept of "safe sex" be rejected, and that – despite overwhelming evidence to the contrary – condoms could not prevent transmission of the virus.

Almost thirty years into the AIDS epidemic, in 2009, Pope Benedict XVI stated (in the context of a program in Africa) that condom distribution actually increases the likelihood of contracting AIDS.

It wasn't until the following year that Pope Benedict XVI – in a statement that required clarification from his office – allowed the possibility that condom use by male prostitutes could be interpreted as a "first assumption of responsibility" – an effort to prevent the spread of the virus.

Many people ignored these statements, just like many Catholics rejected the Church's teachings on birth control. But the damage was done. The spiritual leaders of over a billion people had the opportunity to be not just good fundraisers for their ministries to those already infected – they had the chance to use their influence to save lives.

From the beginning, those who were not directly impacted by AIDS felt free to stand in judgment of those who were. Elton John, in *Love is the Cure: On Life, Loss and the End of AIDS*, remembers:

> Jerry Falwell, the founder of the Moral Majority and a key ally of President Reagan, said that "homosexuals are violating the laws of nature. God establishes all of nature's laws. When a person ignores these laws there is a price to pay."

When the religious right could no longer ignore the complexities of the virus, their attitude evolved: Oh, wait, you have AIDS and you're not a gay man? Then you must've done something else to deserve it used drugs, slept around, lied about it. You're a baby? Well, your mother's the one who's sentenced you to an early death. And if she's infected, too, well…serves her right.

But then came the political conventions of 1992. It was odd: each one gave a prime-time slot to a person living with HIV/AIDS. What was even stranger was that they were both privileged white women.

Elisabeth Glaser, who would die two years later, gave an impassioned speech at the Democratic convention. She was infected via transfusion after giving birth to her daughter, Ariel, who had already died from AIDS when her mother spoke at the convention.

"For me, this is not politics. This is a crisis of caring," she told her largely sympathetic audience.

A month later, at the Republican convention in Houston, Mary Fisher, who was infected by her husband, spoke in her role as an AIDS activist. Her message was a little more blunt: "We cannot love justice and ignore prejudice."

Bigotry and hysteria created as much suffering as AIDS did. People were so focused on blaming the victims that there was no time for compassion, prevention, treatment, research. It was more important for people to feel morally superior. Many years and thousands of lives were wasted while smug, ignorant people shouted curses at a sick twelve-year-old boy from Kokomo, Indiana and others like him.

In the Beginning, Friends Learned a New Alphabet

GRID (Gay-Related Immune Deficiency)

PCP (Pneumocystis Pneumonia)

ARC (AIDS-Related Complex)

OI (Opportunistic Infection)

HTLV/HTLV III (Human T-Lymphotropic Virus, the original name for HIV)

PEPFAR (President's Emergency Plan for AIDS Relief)

PWA/PLWA (People With AIDS/People Living With AIDS)

AZT (the first powerful medication to treat HIV)

KS (Kaposi's Sarcoma)

HIV (Human Immunodeficiency Virus)

AIDS (Acquired Immune Deficiency Syndrome)

PEP (Post-Exposure Prophylaxis)

PrEP (Pre-Exposure Prophylaxis)

As often happens when you are thrown into the alternate universe of a serious medical condition, you have a steep learning curve.

You and your family must learn procedures and treatments and theories and strategies and protocols, whether you want to or not.

For those diagnosed with AIDS, that often means you and your friends, not family, because family ties are often one of the first casualties.

We are a very judgmental society, at least here in the US, and that mindset often permeates even our own families. It wasn't just the disease itself that led families to turn their backs. It was the added stigma of homosexuality (or prostitution or drug abuse). The diagnosis was considered a reflection on the family, a bad one. So many felt justified in abandoning one of their own.

We are quicker to blame victims of disease than the disease itself. We believe ourselves superior in some way to people who are sick because we judge them to be stupid, weak or morally deficient. We feel especially good about ourselves when we can quote Bible verses or local laws to support our position.

Different diseases carry their own stigma. Diagnosed with lung cancer? Well, you shouldn't have smoked. Diagnosed with diabetes or heart disease? Well, you should've lost weight. Diagnosed with AIDS? Oh, where to begin with the criticism?

As Elinor Burkett put it so eloquently in *The Gravest Show on Earth: America in the Age of AIDS,* "AIDS never got a chance to be simply a disease."

This was different, from the start. This was something new and mysterious and terrifying. And friends made all the difference.

Why Friends Mattered – And Still Do

The early days of the AIDS epidemic – even now to a lesser degree – saw shocking expressions of hate and fear. When you add AIDS to the already-volatile issue of homosexuality, there are bound to be casualties.

I remember going to the AIDS ward at Illinois Masonic Medical Center to visit someone I'd met at one of the AIDS housing programs in Chicago. He was young, blonde, attractive; or rather, he had been when I first met him. Now, at 20, he was hospitalized, his body retaining fluid and swelling almost before your eyes.

He'd left instructions for what he wanted done when he died: cremation, no religious ceremony, just his friends in attendance. His family had shunned him because he was gay, and refused to visit him now that he was dying.

Later his caregivers and friends did have a ceremony for him – releasing white balloons after a few words of remembrance. It was all we could do. The day after he died, his family finally appeared to claim his body. They took him back downstate, held a funeral mass and buried him. His friends were not invited.

This was not an unusual story. In Dwight Okita's remembrance that was part of the excellent 2011 "AIDS@30" series in *Windy City Times*, he remembers with great affection his friend Jimmi B.

> I keep his last name hidden behind a single initial because his mother would have preferred it that way. I'm not sure if she is still living, but I know she did not accept her son's orientation. She blamed Jimmi's gay friends for making him gay, for giving him the gay disease, for taking her beloved son so far away from her that she could never again hear her sweet son's laugh…his mother had a small, private funeral, and did not invite his friends.

The toll on friends was – and continues to be – a heavy one. In preparation for this book, I asked a random group of people how many friends they had lost to AIDS over the years. The answers varied:

> None, yet.

> Maybe a dozen, but only two were really close.

> Well, I virtually know no one of my ilk from back then. Very few, if any, survived.

> A significant number (well over 200), partially because of what I do (work in an AIDS-service organization)

The late activist and author of *The Celluloid Closet*, Vito Russo, gave an especially poignant answer in the Academy Award-winning documentary *Common Threads: Stories From the Quilt*:

> I met a 32-year old guy who told me all his friends are dead. All he had were acquaintances left.

I stopped counting at eleven, and if that sounds like a strange number to remember, there's a reason: back when I was a fundraiser, someone I knew died of AIDS every week for eleven weeks in a row. There are more; five come to mind immediately. But that's a list I'm not interested in updating.

Playwright and AIDS activist Larry Kramer did keep a list in the beginning of the epidemic. He stopped early on, in 1985, when the list reached 200.

But he only stopped recording the names in his notebook. He continued to collect obituaries, or pieces of paper where he scribbled a name, and tossed them into a box. In *Reports From the Holocaust: The Story of an AIDS Activist*, Kramer explains in painful detail how he organized the names onto three-by-five cards, alphabetizing and annotating each one. Even the long-time activist was shocked to realize the final count was nearly five hundred. A year later, Kramer added ninety more names to the list.

Friends are important for many reasons, but never so much as at the beginning of the AIDS epidemic. Straight and gay, they bore the responsibility of advocacy and caregiving. They became family, when families abandoned the dying. They responded to the pandemic in ways we often see in the wake of a tragedy, be it a natural disaster, 9/11, or a mass shooting.

Illinois State Rep. Greg Harris (D-13th) spoke to *Windy City Times* in their "AIDS@30" series about just that response:

> We saw our friends getting sick and dying around us. The government was ignoring them. There were no community institutions to help them. The philanthropic community and the corporate community – this was something that wasn't on their radars at the time.
>
> If you look at all the organizations that are now big institutions – big buildings and big staffs – back then it was a bunch of people sitting around kitchen tables trying to figure this out. There was no network of primary care; there was no network of legal-assistance people; and there was no place to get food or pastoral care.

Thousands of organizations were started around the country and fell into three basic categories:

- Some were direct service organizations. These were the ones that provided for the basic, and sometimes unique, needs of those already infected. What patients needed were things as critical as food and housing and as new as legal support against discrimination. People were losing their apartments and their jobs because they had AIDS.

- Second were fundraising organizations. Most corporate and private foundations were not funding AIDS services in any way. Eventually corporations began supporting events, in order to benefit from marketing exposure. Private foundations could be picky, concerned (with good reason) about the proliferation of new organizations resulting in needless duplication of services. AIDS-specific foundations sprouted, including AIDS Foundation of Chicago and Broadway Cares/Equity Fights AIDS.

- Lastly were organizations that focused on the often-thankless job of prevention. They were the ones organizing needle exchanges, in violation of local laws. They were the ones handing out free condoms at bars and Gay Pride parades. They were the ones banned from disseminating educational materials to schools, and ridiculed for trying to shut down the baths.

They all had two things in common: they were created by people – mostly in the gay community – who were desperate to help their friends (and often, themselves) stay alive. And they would serve as models for future grassroots response to a medical crisis.

Friends were thrust into the role of caregiver. There was really no choice. Their families, even if nearby, often chose to abandon them.

There were two reasons why AIDS housing programs were necessary. First, people were being kicked out of their apartments when their diagnosis became known, or losing their homes because they could no longer support themselves. They couldn't even go on disability, because according to the Social Security Administration, AIDS didn't fit their criteria.

The other reason was that they had nowhere else to go. People with AIDS were denied admission to hospitals, because administrators didn't want theirs to be known as "the AIDS hospital" and become a dumping ground. Nursing homes were established for the elderly, or, in some cases, severely disabled. They were not equipped to accept – nor did they want – people with AIDS.

Caregivers – whether friends or paid workers from social service agencies – burned linens, bleached their hands and required visitors to wear hospital gowns and masks. Fear drove behavior and policies, especially in the early days, because so little was known.

Working on the front lines every day, those of us in the AIDS community did what we could to protect ourselves – not from the virus, but from the emotional devastation of losing friends. As Trudy Ring, who was a volunteer at Chicago House when I worked there, put it:

> I didn't want to work in one of the residences, as some volunteers did – I feared I'd get too emotionally involved with the residents, and hence depressed.

For Trudy, volunteering in the office doing clerical and fundraising projects – that worked. But it only worked until she became friends with those around her.

Consciously or not, I hoped I could do what she attempted: distance herself from really close contact to protect herself emotionally. But in the end, it didn't work.

It's hard for most people to imagine losing so many friends. It was the same after 9/11. Survivors lost neighbors and co-workers; the guy who sold them their morning paper and the waitress who greeted them as a regular; the people they saw in the elevator whose names they never knew. But all of them died at once, on one terrible morning. Their suffering was over quickly, rather than happening over weeks, months, years.

Bill Hayes describes what it was like in *AIDS@30: A Time Capsule* on the *New York Review of Books* blog:

> Faces of the dead surfaced weekly in the *Bay Area Reporter*, a local gay newspaper that published obituaries with photos of men who had recently

died. Picking up a copy, I would instinctively open first to this section; it filled two pages or more. I always recognized someone I had known, danced, slept or worked out with, aware that, in a barely different narrative, one of the pictures could have been my own.

It's only recently that I've heard anyone speak of survivor guilt in the AIDS community. It seems a natural result of having lived within this world for three decades. But especially for gay men of a certain age, AIDS is like a sword of Damocles hanging over their heads. They're spared, but they're not really certain why.

Support groups addressing the unique physical and psychological needs of these long-term survivors are finally being formed.

For those who have lost friends to AIDS, the losses are ongoing, relentless. At the height of the epidemic, you might lose a friend/acquaintance a week; maybe more. Now the numbers here in the US have slowed down. Now it might be one every few months.

But remember: these losses have been piling up for over thirty years.

Thirty years.

Some people have kept count. Dick Uyvari kept a list of bowlers in the LGBT bowling leagues in Chicago. The list dwindled from a total of over 800 in the mid-80s to less than 700 by 1992: one of every eight was gone.

Middle-aged gay men – many of whom did not expect to live through the 80s and 90s – find themselves with few friends their own age, if any.

Elton John can give you a pretty close number of friends

he's lost: maybe 80. He built a chapel on his property. There he has a plaque for each of his friends who have died, many from AIDS.

If there has been an upside of AIDS, it's a new appreciation of friendships, both gay and straight. In a reflective moment in *Reports from the Holocaust: Diary of an AIDS Activist*, Larry Kramer considers the changing nature of gay men's friendships. Instead of taking years to mature and deepen, friendships developed quickly. There, in the battlefield, there was no time to think long-term.

Now, in the fourth decade of the epidemic, others are sharing their experiences. Recent books and documentaries focus on both the history of the epidemic and needs of long-term survivors. Those histories are largely those told by white gay men in specific urban areas (New York and San Francisco).

The experiences of people of color, trans men and trans women are just beginning to be included. Oral histories such as ACT UP Oral History Project and Story Corps have been instrumental in bringing many of these stories to light. The absence of straight women in most narratives inspired me to write my next book, *Fag Hags, Divas and Moms: The Legacy of Straight Women in the AIDS Community*.

There is no definitive history of the AIDS epidemic. It's impossible, though there are many brilliant films and books out there. But all of them share one desire, to honor friends for their contributions.

Silence=Death –
How ACT UP Changed Everything

> "ACT UP is a diverse, non-partisan group of individuals, united in anger and committed to direct action to end the AIDS crisis."

There are many things we take for granted, when it comes to catastrophic diseases.

As a society, we now feel comfortable educating ourselves about drugs, procedures and treatments, especially on the internet.

We sign petitions to demand funding for our particular medical concern.

We join organizations devoted to educating and advocating for funding, treatment and cures.

We demand clinical trials that are not double blind.

We testify before local, state and federal governments about the need for increased funding, and contact our lawmakers.

We expect drugs to be approved by the FDA in a timely manner.

We support celebrities who support our favorite cause.

We wear ribbons of varying colors – red, pink, teal, grey.

We buy products sold with the promise that "a portion of the sale" will go to our favorite cause.

When you do any of these things, you owe a debt to ACT UP.

Before the AIDS epidemic forced people to become instant authorities on medical treatments and fierce advocates for funding none of these things were commonplace. In fact, some of them just weren't done. The 60's and 70's were full of public demonstrations against war and racism. But demonstrating about clinical trials and treatment access? That was very new.

"Don't practice medicine without a license," my late father used to say. He was not of a generation that self-diagnosed or questioned doctors.

But AIDS forever changed the relationship of ordinary people to the medical establishment, and its supporters: religious institutions, charitable foundations and a myriad of government agencies.

The AIDS community had no choice. Life expectancy was measured in weeks or months. There was no known effective treatment for the rare AIDS-related infections, viruses or cancers. No one was sure how it was transmitted or who was truly at risk.

There was no choice but to confront every part of the establishment – government, medicine, drug manufacturers, insurance companies – because their lives, and the lives of their friends, were at stake.

There aren't a lot of things that will try your patience like knowing that you or your friends are dying and the clock is ticking. You have no time to waste on people who operate on "this is the way it's always been done" basis.

With the AIDS epidemic, the status quo didn't work anymore. That meant a new way of dealing with health crises was needed.

What complicated this situation was the discrimination against gay men that was already ingrained in our society. Most people were simply not inclined to help them. As the disease spread, infecting women, children and minorities, the fear of infection trumped compassion, even for the "innocent" victims.

What to do? People were dying – in their homes, in hospital hallways, on the street. Drugs that were sold over the counter in other countries required years of clinical trials to be approved in the US. Attempts at prevention – needle exchange programs, free condoms – were blocked time and again by conservative Christian legislators whose condemnation of the gay "lifestyle" literally sentenced people to death.

The people who started ACT UP in New York City in 1987 did what people do when faced with a crisis or injustice: they took to the streets – sometimes literally.

The AIDS Coalition To Unleash Power was not the typical advocacy group. But then, there weren't advocacy groups then. Their tactics, fueled by a desperate race against the clock, enraged and motivated the country.

One aspect of the beginnings of ACT UP was the complication of class and gender. The gay men initially affected by AIDS tended to be white, financially secure and often closeted. As long as the issue wasn't gay rights, they were secure in the knowledge that The System worked as well for them as it did for straight white men.

So when AIDS began to spread, they did not expect to lose their jobs, be evicted from their homes or find that their doctors were not able to provide an accurate diagnosis, let alone the willingness to treat them. They did not expect to go from sexual revolutionaries (remember Gay Liberation?) to dying patients in a short time. They did not expect to be forced out of the closet to confront the twin prejudices against those with AIDS and gay men in general. They expected to be treated with respect, their demands met quickly.

It was a shock when that didn't happen.

Some of them saw enough horrific deaths to know that everything in their world had changed. They quickly realized that the government's insistence on the need to move slowly on AIDS made no sense.

The FDA insisted on adhering to a process of drug testing (only on white gay men – no minorities, women or children were included for years) that included double-blind clinical trials and the use of placebos: a process that could drag on as long as ten years. They resisted reacting to this new AIDS threat more quickly, even though some of the drugs they were testing were already being sold over the counter in other countries.

The AIDS community's anger was justified: Local, state and federal authorities mobilized quickly in 1976, when the first large outbreak of Legionnaire's disease killed thirty-four people in Philadelphia. Likewise, in 1982, it took only seven people killed in the Tylenol murders to spark a nationwide recall of the painkiller and fast action from all levels of government. But that kind of response wasn't happening with AIDS, because it was happening to a group that many felt deserved to be punished.

But that kind of response wasn't happening with AIDS,

because it was mostly happening to a group that many felt deserved to be punished. The numbers are hard to grasp:

In 1981, 385 Americans died of AIDS.

By 1988, the total had risen to 55,388.

In the first seven years, the number dead in the US neared the total for the almost two-decade long Vietnam War (58,220). But for those with AIDS, there was no cease-fire.

And so ACT UP was born.

Their tactics were never subtle, but they did things that we now take for granted, including testifying on Capitol Hill and holding demonstrations at churches, government buildings and drug companies.

They lay down in the center aisle of St. Patrick's Cathedral, disrupting Sunday mass, in the presence of the Cardinal and the mayor, Ed Koch, while 7,000 demonstrators filled 5th Avenue outside. They shouted down drug company CEO's and politicians in their offices, during press conferences, and in public. They covered conservative Congressman Jesse Helms' house with a gigantic condom.

And they did what we all had to do: self-educate. One of the most interesting scenes in the documentary *How to Survive A Plague* shows an ACT UP member handing out a glossary of medical terms at one of their meetings. "Learn them," was the directive. They weren't just going to be a group of angry people. They were going to be a well-educated group of angry people who could argue the merits of various drugs, therapies and clinical trial protocols with those who developed and controlled them.

And they did something else: they filmed *everything*. They preserved organizational meetings (the nonprofit equivalent of watching sausage made) by multiple members holding those awkwardly large camcorders. All demonstrations were taped. I couldn't imagine watching videos of the early meetings of nonprofits I've helped found. Why did ACT UP do this, from the very beginning?

United in Anger – which, like *How to Survive a Plague*, chronicles the early history of ACT UP – provided the explanation of why they documented their actions so relentlessly: to control the message. Rather than rely on what the mainstream (and even gay) media chose to report, ACT UP's media-savvy members taped everything themselves. They made videotapes and sent them to media outlets around the world. They ensured that their message got out accurately.

One example: the AIDS ward at Cook County Hospital in Chicago was one of the best in the country…if you were a man. Women – assuming they were accurately diagnosed with AIDS – were spread throughout the hospital. The media were unaware of the one and only reason why this was happening: there were only men's restrooms on the AIDS floor and the County Board refused to spend $1,000 to install one for women. ACT UP threatened an action and alerted the media. The money was approved within 24 hours.

People in power – politicians, drug company executives, media, doctors and researchers – had never been confronted like this.

The civil rights movement of the 1960's targeted all aspects of society – from voter registration to housing to educational access – to expose and change systemic discrimination. What ACT UP did was similarly broad. But they added the interconnectedness of government policies and medical treatment.

The fact that ACT UP members could speak knowledgeably and passionately about drug protocols and the impact of specific legislation changed the discourse and the relationship between the powers that be and the general public forever.

Everyone who advocates for a particular health cause, be it breast cancer or autism, owes a debt of gratitude to ACT UP for leading the way.

The Quilt and Grieving

Near my cubicle at Chicago House, where I was the Development Director from 1989-90, was a table with a book on it. There were other books, but one was always on top. It was *The Quilt: Stories from the Names Project* by Cindy Ruskin.

The AIDS Memorial Quilt was two years old, but already was comprised of hundreds of panels, each made in loving tribute to a person (or persons) who died of AIDS.

I remember looking down at the cover that displayed several panels and thinking "Gee, he looks familiar." I couldn't place him. He had that perfect moustache and artfully tousled hair so many gay men adopted at the time. I opened the book to the cover illustration credits, and there was David Aurand's name. That's how I found out he was dead.

We weren't close; we'd done shows together in college, and I hadn't seen him since then. But I'd been out of touch with other gay men I knew, so I started looking up names in the index. I was relieved when I didn't find one in particular. But I did find his brother.

The Names Project AIDS Memorial Quilt – usually referred to only as "the Quilt" – is a unique response to loss. In some ways, it's the polar opposite of ACT UP.

> The Quilt was conceived in November of 1985 by long-time San Francisco gay rights activist Cleve Jones. Since the 1978 assassinations of gay San Francisco Supervisor Harvey Milk and Mayor George Moscone, Jones had helped organize the annual candlelight march honoring these men. While planning the 1985 march, he learned that over 1,000 San Franciscans had been lost to AIDS. He asked each of his fellow marchers to write on placards the names of friends and loved ones who had died of AIDS. At the end of the march, Jones and others stood on ladders taping these placards to the walls of the San Francisco Federal Building. The wall of names looked like a patchwork quilt. (from the Names Project website)

When people started writing names on the placards that night, they would only put a first name and last initial. AIDS was still in the closet, and there was shame in identifying those who had died from it. Eventually, some added last names. People in the crowd began to identify men they knew who had died.

Though the Quilt's beginning was rooted in the gay community, surprising partners came forth to support it, like the Junior League. The city of Torino, Italy, underwrote its display. While quilting is a uniquely American folk art, there are traditions indigenous to other countries that are comparable. So the Quilt has traveled not just around the US, but as far away as Indonesia, South Africa and Guatemala.

Since 1987, 18 million people have visited the Quilt, which was last displayed in its entirety in 1996. At 1.3 million square feet, too large to unfold in any one place, it now includes over 48,000 panels with 94,000 names. It travels in sections, for World AIDS Day commemorations, conferences and other events.

Reading the biographies of participants in the 2012 Smithsonian Folklife Festival's "Creativity and Crisis – Unfolding the AIDS Memorial Quilt" exhibit, is to understand how friends fit into the AIDS epidemic:

> Cleve Jones, co-founder of the Names Project Foundation made the first panel for a friend.
>
> Gert McMillan, Quilt Production Manager and "Keeper of the Quilt" got involved when many of her friends died of AIDS in the early 80s.
>
> Chili Crane, current warehouse manager for The Quilt, recently started work on a panel in memory of a friend who died a few years ago.
>
> Roddy Williams, director of operations at the Name Project Foundation has been working with the Quilt since 2003, but became more emotionally involved in 2006 when he lost one of his best friends to AIDS.

For many people, the act of coming together to make a quilt panel was healing. Everyone there – sewing, cutting, designing – was going through the same experience. All were grieving for someone, and many were grieving for multiple friends. The process of making the panels could be compared to group therapy for those who need to work through their grief.

"Anger and spray paint don't mix very well," explained Clarissa Crabtree, who has worked with the Quilt for more than twenty years, at the Smithsonian Festival. The Quilt tended to attract people who were less confrontational, less likely to be angry while they sewed and glued and painted their panels.

Visiting the Quilt – seeing the panel of someone you knew and loved – is like visiting a cemetery. Volunteers unfold and smooth down the panels in a solemn ritual. Other volunteers are available at the showings, to help you find a panel and give you comfort. For some who create or visit, it's the only tangible memory of their friend.

On the occasions when I've seen the Quilt displayed, I've checked ahead of time to find out if the panels of people I knew would be there. But I always feel tense when I walk around, afraid I'll be surprised to see the name of someone I didn't know had died of AIDS.

Thousands of names, thousands of panels, commemorating the lives of people who died from this virus: it's a gentle, respectful tribute. And it's not without its critics.

Early on, the Quilt – like the seemingly endless candlelight vigils – was viewed as a vehicle for grief: public, but non-confrontational. At worst, its critics viewed it as ineffectual and defeatist.

Perhaps not surprisingly, the relationship of the Quilt and ACT UP is a complicated one. In *Moving Politics: Emotion and ACT UP's Fight Against AIDS*, Deborah Gould succinctly defines the tension:

Rather than regarding the quilt as a memorial to gay men and others who had died, ACT UP suggested it be viewed as a chronicle of murder that necessitated a forceful activist response.

Indeed, at the October, 1988 Quilt display in Washington, ACT UP handed out flyers that read:

Show your **anger** to the people who helped make the Quilt possible: our **government!**

Both responses are understandable. The Quilt was needed as a way to express grief. Remember: early in the epidemic, most funeral homes would not take bodies of people who died of AIDS. "Normal" funerals were rare: even churches refused to hold services for them. Memorial services after cremation were typical. Cemetery burials were rare, with unintended consequences: Ryan White's gravestone was vandalized four times in the year after his death.

The AIDS community was forced to create new ways to grieve.

ACT UP used the Quilt, but didn't abuse it: When both groups descended on Washington in 1992, ACT UP marchers were silent as they passed the Quilt display on the National Mall. Once past, they resumed their chanting as they headed up to the White House, where they threw the ashes of their loved ones over the fence.

Both groups – the Name Project and ACT UP – describe their intent that day in the same way: "Bringing the dead to your door."

I believe that the AIDS community needed – and continues to need – both the Quilt and ACT UP. Channeling grief into anger (a much-used description of ACT UP) is appropriate and necessary. But skipping over grief in order to do that rarely works. Eventually the anger fades – because it's been resolved, or because you're exhausted – and grief bubbles up again. And that makes the catharsis the Quilt provides a necessary one.

When I was at the Smithsonian Folkways Festival, I realized pretty quickly that something was missing, at least for me. I'd walked around the Quilt and seen panels that are famous for their message, like:

> "Don't let my epitaph be that I died of red tape."

There were no panels of people I'd known on display, which frankly, was a relief. As I walked around in triple digit heat, something began to rise up in me. At first I thought I was just crabby from the swamp-like humidity. But it wasn't that. I couldn't put my finger on it, until I was sitting in on a panel discussion about the Quilt and asked the following:

> "No one's angry anymore. Why isn't anyone angry?"

Some panelists and audience members nodded in agreement. Gert McMullin eagerly admitted her anger, even after all these years:

> "I use anger as food. It gives me energy. I want to be angry because it gives me the energy to deal."

Clarissa, on the other hand, preferred to think about the positives:

> "How would they want me to remember them, to live my life?"

Mike Smith and Cleve Jones weren't thinking about 25 years down the road when they started the Quilt. They were only looking for a way to honor their friends in that moment.

Yes, it's great it's still going after all these years. It's great that there is such a powerful visual reminder of the toll of not only the AIDS virus, but of prejudice and indifference.

But it's still growing, and I wish to God we didn't need it.

Guilt/Sainthood by Association

When I was working in the AIDS community, I used to cringe when people asked what I did for a living. My reply that I raised money for AIDS-service organizations was met with one of three reactions:

Really? Tell me more about what you do. (Honestly, I rarely heard that.)

Ewwww... (Some variation of this was most likely.)

Oh, you're so wonderful to do that. (The most annoying of all.)

I didn't date much when I was doing that work. Straight men tended to run the other way when I told them who my clients were.

Occasionally, someone – often a closeted gay man – would want to know more about my work. I was always willing to explain, and often wound up making referrals.

But the reality of my job was more complex. The volunteer director at a large AIDS-service organization in Los Angeles told me:

> I don't consider myself more compassionate than anyone else or more informed than anyone else but automatically, I become the noble person taking on the good fight. In some cases, I become taboo because I represent the disease to them. In other areas, it's assumption after assumption. For instance, you must be HIV-positive or you're so compassionate because of what you do. It can become quite tiring. I do what I do because I enjoy what I do. I wish there was no need to do it but it's my choice. I just get tired of people filtering it through some perspective of martyrdom or sainthood.

I raised money over the years for different types of organizations – educational, performing arts, social services – but only my work with AIDS elicited those kinds of responses.

Perhaps I shouldn't have been annoyed. I made a conscious decision to get involved because I wanted to make a difference, no matter how small. And isn't that why we all get involved in causes that are important to us? But this particular cause – with its attendant homophobia, discrimination and hysteria – was unique.

I didn't feel special, or that I was worthy of attention. I felt like an outsider; like I lived in some kind of alternate universe where my friends were dying and the rest of the world didn't care.

The Other Kind of Guilt

Not everyone responded to the AIDS crisis with action. In the early days, a lot more gay men were closeted. No matter their HIV status, they didn't necessarily jump at the chance to become involved.

They had a lot to lose – support of their families, jobs, housing, friends – if they chose this time to come out. Even if they didn't have the virus, people would assume they did.

So they wrote checks. I had a donor at Chicago House who wrote a generous check every month. I kept his name in the top drawer of my desk, a constant reminder that he did not want to receive event invitations. I assumed at the time that he just didn't want to get a lot of mail, but now I wonder if he may have preferred not going public with his support.

Making financial contributions was a way of supporting the cause – often anonymously – without shouting it to the world. It's not that these men weren't already affected by the AIDS crisis; they were. But that was the limit they set on involvement. Perhaps that was all they could muster.

For those on the front lines of the war against AIDS, for those who numbered their dead friends in the dozens, if not hundreds, that limited participation was a crime.

At his friend Jeff Schmalz's memorial service on December 7, 1993, Larry Kramer let loose on the other mourners, and rightly so. Looking out at the crowd, he saw people who dutifully showed up at these services, but did nothing to use their financial or political power to help stop the epidemic. To those who had been on the front lines since the beginning, that inaction was nothing less than unforgiveable.

Individuals and corporations were slow to come around, if at all. Major newspapers reported deaths as "after a long illness" rather than from AIDS, even into the second decade of the epidemic.

In *Love is the Cure: On Life, Love and the End of AIDS*, Elton John's memoir about the AIDS epidemic, he blames his behavior in the 80s on his all-consuming addictions:

> I'm deeply ashamed that I didn't do more about AIDS back then. My friends were dying all around me, and with few exceptions I failed to act. I gave some money to foundations. I performed at AIDS benefits. I helped [Ryan White and his family]. I recorded a song called "That's What Friends Are For" with Gladys Knight, Stevie Wonder, and Dionne Warwick; the proceeds from that single went to the American Foundation for AIDS Research (amfAR). But the fact is that I was a gay man in the 80s who didn't

march. I didn't give the time or effort that I easily could have, and should have, to fight AIDS and support those who had it.

I don't think anyone argues with his self-assessment. The important thing, then, is what he did to overcome that guilt.

It wasn't easy. But ultimately it was his friendship with Ryan White – unlikely though genuine – that has guided him. In reading his book, it is no exaggeration to say that Elton John turned his life around – confronting his multiple addictions and finding a new purpose – because of that friendship.

> I'm here today because of Ryan. He inspired me to fix my life and start my AIDS foundation. He continues to inspire me each and every day. I know that he looked up to me, and the thought of disappointing him now, even though he is long gone, makes me shudder. I try to honor his memory by living the way he would want me to live, by being the person he thought that I was.

What has guided Elton John is what guides many of us after the death of a friend: the desire to give back, to make the world a better place, as they made it for us.

The Glamor Quotient

Like other fundraising professionals, I had my wardrobe: suits for meetings with donors or going to memorial services, jeans for setting up events, cocktail dresses for black-tie dinners.

For those in the AIDS community, our social lives revolved around two things: funerals and fundraisers.

It was, in a perverse way, glamorous. By 1990, money was starting to flow: from the government, foundations, corporations, individuals. That meant lots of events: walks, house tours, dances, black-tie dinners, cocktail parties, concerts, drag shows. There were fundraising events every night of the week. Looking back, it feels like they were all set to music: mostly disco and Broadway show tunes.

One of the most popular songs of the day was "Wind Beneath My Wings", sung by Bette Midler in *Beaches*. A beautiful testimony to friendship, it became the AIDS national anthem, at least in my mind. It was played at most of the fundraisers and memorial services I attended, leaving not a dry eye in the house. After a while, though, it set my teeth on edge. When I got married, my father wanted it to be his first dance with me at the reception. I refused. I hated to say no, because he loved the song. But it was too damn sad, for me and my friends. So it was more than ironic that years later, it was the only song we played at his funeral. If I never hear it again, it'll be too soon.

Until I worked in the AIDS community, black-tie dinners tended to be stodgy, boring evenings redeemed only by free-flowing alcohol. But now I looked forward to them. Produced by the gay community, there was a frenzied competition to raise the bar on every aspect: décor, food, entertainment and fundraising goals. And there was always a good looking guy who was willing and eager to dance.

It wasn't unusual to be entertained by Broadway or Hollywood stars, nor to count the evening's take in the millions. They were elaborate, perfectly executed productions. In ballrooms around the country, the stigma of AIDS did not exist.

These events were not just an opportunity to raise much-needed money to support those living with AIDS, conduct research into treatments and a cure, or support prevention efforts. They were an escape.

For a few hours on a Saturday night, we could dress up and forget about what was happening outside that hotel ballroom. We could dine on gourmet food, drink premium liquor, bid on fairy-tale-worthy auction items, and be entertained by the likes of Michael Feinstein, Elizabeth Taylor, Angela Lansbury or Elton John.

I wonder sometimes if AIDS would have become worldwide

news if it had hit a different demographic first and hardest (though it did, eventually). What if the virus was spreading only among IV-drug users or prostitutes, anonymous groups of people with no public advocates? What if it had started in sub-Saharan Africa and then made its way to the US?

But from early on – in part, by virtue of the number of gay men in those professions – AIDS had a celebrity quotient. The Artists with AIDS website today lists over 1,800 people in the visual and performing arts who died from AIDS. Household names were in the news, not because of their work, but their HIV status:

Liberace, performer

Scott McPherson, playwright

Michael Bennett, director

Rudolf Nureyev, dancer

Keith Haring, artist

Rock Hudson, actor

Robert Joffrey, choreographer

Freddy Mercury, singer and composer

Whether or not they admitted beforehand that they were gay, these were men whose accomplishments in the arts were world-renowned. We were fans. We bought tickets to their performances and watched their movies. In the case of Magic Johnson (who revealed his HIV status in 1991 and is still alive), we watched him play basketball.

So when the big, high-ticket fundraising events were produced, it was their friends who attended and performed.

Not everyone, of course, had hundreds or thousands of dollars for a ticket to these events, so smaller events flourished. AIDS walks (typically 10K) popped up in cities large and small. Gay bars donated cover charges, or kept donation cans in a prominent location (sometimes next to the bowl of free condoms).

And then there were the red ribbons.

In June, 1991, the Artists' Caucus of Visual AIDS (an organization of visual artists who created "A Day Without Art") entered into a partnership with Broadway Cares/Equity Fights AIDS (BC/EFA). That year, at the 45th annual Tony Awards, actor Jeremy Irons was the first person to wear a red ribbon and publicly acknowledge the symbolism of supporting those living with HIV/AIDS. It didn't take long for the red ribbon to become an international symbol of AIDS awareness.

As with many good ideas, this one fell victim to commercialization. It's a simple gesture of solidarity and support to wear a red ribbon on your lapel. It becomes something crass when a company makes it not with grosgrain but with cubic zirconia and offers it for sale in a limited edition, "a portion of which will be donated to AIDS charities". Because Visual AIDS deliberately did not copyright the idea, anyone could (and still can) use it any way they wanted.

There were a lot of fundraising scams out there, once it was clear there was money to be had. Some were without malice: events run by well-intentioned people who were poor organizers. Some of them were like the example above, where someone would take a lovely idea like the Visual AIDS red ribbon, and use it as a marketing tool. Does a promise that "twenty-five cents from the sale of each lipstick goes to AIDS research" make you want to buy it? Should it? And how do you know for sure the company will pass along that quarter?

Maybe because of my experiences in the AIDS community,

maybe because I was a fundraiser for a lot of years, but these kinds of sales pitches make me run the other way.

Many cities hold AIDS walks, usually in the fall. But there's one day every year marked around the world: December 1, World AIDS Day.

I was in London on December 1, 1988. At the curtain call of the Sherlock Holmes play I attended, Jeremy Brett, who played the lead, made a speech. He announced that it was the first World AIDS Day, and ushers would be taking donations for AIDS organizations in London. When he finished, ushers walked up and down the aisles, each carrying a can for patrons to put money into. I put a couple pounds in, and filed away the idea for future reference.

A year later, at Chicago House, I sent out teams of volunteers to Off-Loop theatres to make curtain speeches and solicit donations for our programs. I figured it was a good idea: it cost us nothing, and drew attention to this new "holiday."

For years, Broadway Cares/Equity Fights AIDS has run similar but greatly expanded program to raise money for their programs and grants. Running a full six weeks around World AIDS Day (and also in the spring), most Broadway shows participate. In addition to collecting donations, they sell autographed programs and memorabilia from the plays, as well as photo opportunities with the performers. In 2011, these efforts raised two-thirds of the $9.3 million BC/EFA distributed to over 500 AIDS service organizations around the country and the Actors Fund.

Long after the face of AIDS changed, the arts community continues to support the cause, in sometimes flashy but always deeply committed, ways.

No Big Deal Anymore, Right?

In the fourth decade of the AIDS epidemic (and I can't believe I just typed those words), what's changed? What's the same?

Doneley Meris, founder and Executive Director of HIV Arts Network in New York City, told me about the changes – for good and bad – that he sees, particularly in relation to the LGBT community.

In 1981, no one anticipated a day when people with AIDS would live long enough to die from "normal" diseases, like cancer or heart disease. No one imagined that the right drug 'cocktail' would prolong your life indefinitely. No one believed survival rates would be measured in decades rather than weeks. No one even assumed a future need for senior services in the gay community.

What struck me the most about our conversation was the generational disconnect, due in some part to those medical advances. As great as these new drugs are, they've had a dangerous, unintended consequence.

Older gay men, those who lived through the past 30 years of the epidemic, now watch a younger generation that not only considers an AIDS diagnosis to be "no big deal", but who sometimes seek out infection. They place ads in gay papers looking for men who will infect them with the AIDS virus, so they can qualify for free housing and other benefits.

Similarly, a gay man on the West Coast told me that some young men intentionally try to get infected because "all the love in the gay community is for men with AIDS." It's seen by these young men as a way to get attention and love, rather than social services.

Even some older men, burned out on decades of safe sex, take risks because they're just tired of it all. In the fourth decade of the epidemic, straight people still don't consider themselves at risk. Those 50 and older – well past the concerns of an unwanted pregnancy – do not have safe sex in mind. But they have the same HIV risk factors as younger people.

And because now it's…no big deal.

For a generation that had become somewhat numb to death, there is no mistaking the anger many of them feel.

Is this why we threw our lovers' ashes at the White House?

Is this why we marched on Congress and the drug companies?

Is this why we cared for and buried dozens of our friends?

So that you can get infected *on purpose*?

The advances in medical treatment and diagnosis have – in the western world – relegated AIDS and HIV to the status of a "chronic" disease. We tout these victories proudly, and press for those treatments to be available and affordable around the world, especially in Africa, where AIDS diagnoses are skyrocketing.

But here in the US…no big deal. I share Larry Kramer's belief that as a society we have decided it's easier to manage AIDS than to address its causes. It's less messy. It's easier to pat ourselves on the back and say "Look how far we've come."

After all, public acceptance of the LGBTQ community is at an all-time high: gay marriage and civil unions are being adopted by more states every year, Don't Ask Don't Tell is history. Openly gay politicians and celebrities are no longer rare. Wearing a red ribbon is no longer a symbol of protest or sign of solidarity. It's just…retro.

I'm pretty sure people don't smoke cigarettes because they want to get lung cancer or heart disease. I'm pretty sure people don't drink too much alcohol in hopes of developing cirrhosis. Why then, are people deliberately infecting themselves with AIDS?

The reasons given above are true, and in the minds of those young men, justified. It's hard enough to fight the Catholic Church's refusal to approve the use of condoms. It's hard enough to fight corrupt governments in Africa and Asia that pocket aid money and let their people die. But how do you fight the idea that deliberately getting infected with AIDS is a good idea?

As Dwayne Carl, author and AIDS activist put it:

> I am angry that there is no sense of urgency about this pandemic. The media and people in general here in the US feel that since it is no longer a death sentence that we don't have to worry about talking about it. [I am] sad, because silently, the rate of

infections nationwide is increasing at alarming rates in every nationality, some more than others.... AIDS is not over...

Out of sight, out of mind. Other crises – economic, political, medical – now command the spotlight. Much of the world has moved on, because AIDS is "manageable." But for those who carry the virus – and those of us who love them – AIDS continues to be something to fight, until that day when it's relegated to history books.

How We Remember Them

The Quilt is a visually stunning, overwhelmingly huge memorial to thousands of men, women and children who have died of AIDS. Too large to display in its entirety any more, sections of it are shipped around the world for World AIDS Day observances.

ACT UP continues to advocate for education, prevention and research, and demand affordable, safe medical treatments for every man, woman and child who needs them.

Broadway Cares/Equity Fights AIDS rallies the theatre community to raise millions of dollars year after year to support the AIDS community.

But there are other ways that people continue to remember their friends lost to AIDS.

Nonprofit organizations around the world, from tiny storefront clinics in impoverished neighborhoods to the United Nations, serve on the front lines of the epidemic:

educating, treating, advocating.

Individuals pour their energies into raising money to support those organizations, through glitzy fundraising events, bike rides and thousands of other appeals.

Some now focus on physical, permanent memorials. In New York City, plans are underway for a small memorial park across from the old St. Vincent's Hospital (which is soon to become luxury condominiums), ground zero in the early fight against AIDS in the West Village.

But there is already a small, quiet memorial in New York, in Hudson River Park between 11th and 12th Streets. It consists only of a curved stone bench on a granite path, cut out of a landscaped knoll at Bank Street. It's a place for contemplation, for remembering.

No names are inscribed, stitched or printed. No one is yelling or chanting. In fact, few people are even aware of this memorial's existence. It's nowhere near as ambitious as the National AIDS Memorial Grove in San Francisco's Golden Gate Park.

In the end, what many of us crave is the quiet, the solitude. We don't need to see names displayed, like the Vietnam Veterans Memorial. We couldn't forget the names of our friends if we wanted to. Their lives and deaths are part of us.

Those friends are remembered by health professionals around the world who work towards a cure and affordable treatment for all.

Those friends are remembered by advocates at all levels of government who believe AIDS is a health issue, not a moral issue, deserving of funding and support.

Those friends are remembered by nonprofit organizations filling in the gaps for people living with AIDS, providing them with housing, food, legal assistance and other social services denied them.

Those friends, finally, are remembered by those of us left behind. We remember them and who we were when we were with them.

I believe they would want us to remember an earlier time before there was such a thing in the world as AIDS: how alive they were, not how much they suffered later. I believe they would want the lucky ones – those with access to the drugs they need to stay alive – to not waste the opportunity denied to them.

They would want us to keep up the good fight: the one where we keep AIDS in the public eye, in the conversation, so that no one takes for granted how far we've come or how far we still have to go.

On World AIDS Day, 2012, I sat in St. Joseph's Church on the north side of Chicago for a service led by my former pastor. Father Pat has been known to give great homilies – my wedding, for one. But that Saturday night he outdid himself. His story was one that follows a familiar pattern: how meeting someone with AIDS changed their perception of the virus.

He was called to the man's expensive home on a genteel, tree-lined street on the Gold Coast to offer prayers. That night, in the early 80s, he learned two important things.

First, that no amount of money could protect you from this new, frightening virus. He was shocked at the man's physical condition, his body wasting away in that beautiful home. And Fr. Pat admitted to being more than a little frightened himself.

Second, he learned of the boundless love that man's friends showed for him. They were his caregivers, taking turns tending to his needs. Even with so little known at the time about how the virus was transmitted, they didn't hesitate to do what was required. "They were the bravest people I'd ever seen," Fr. Pat recalled.

Someday a vaccine and cure for AIDS will finally be found, and it will be relegated to history books like the Black Plague. "Back when people died from AIDS" will begin lectures and textbooks.

When the story of the AIDS epidemic is written (in the past tense) the underlying theme will be of friendship: of the men and women, gay and straight, of all racial and ethnic groups who tended to and buried their friends, who marched and demonstrated and testified, who raised money and awareness – all in the name of their friends.

Maybe you've been involved in the AIDS community, maybe not. Maybe other diseases or issues threaten your friends. But whatever they are, I hope the examples in this book will inspire you to help them and their cause: give money, volunteer your time, educate yourself, spread the word to others.

You don't have to lay down your life for your friend – just give of yourself. And that, after all, is the true meaning of friendship.

On World AIDS Day, 2016, the face of AIDS looked like this:

In the US:

Since June 5, 1981, 1.7 million have been infected with HIV and nearly 650,000 people have died of AIDS and HIV-related illnesses.

There are an estimated 50,000 new infections in the US each year. Women, who typically contract the virus through heterosexual sex, make up 20%, with the infection rate four times higher in African-American women than white women.

In 2010, 31% of new infections occurred among people age 25-34; 26% among people 13-24.

Men who have sex with men account for the majority of HIV/AIDS diagnoses.

African-Americans accounted for 47% of new infections in 2011; the infection rate among Latinos was three times higher than that for whites in 2010.

1.2 million Americans are living with HIV, including an estimated 230,000 who don't know they've been infected.

1/3 of those diagnosed with HIV will develop full-blown AIDS within 1 year of diagnosis.

There has been a 92% decrease in HIV transmission from mother to fetus.

Every year, nearly 17,500 Americans die from AIDS-related causes.

World-wide:

More than 35 million people live with HIV/AIDS.

70% of them live in sub-Saharan Africa including 88% of the world's HIV+ children.

3.3 million of them are under the ages of 15.

Since the beginning of the epidemic, 75 million people have contracted HIV, and nearly 36 million of them have died from HIV-related causes.

(Statistics courtesy of amfAR and UNAIDS)

References:

Burkett, Elinor. *The Gravest Show on Earth: America in the Age of AIDS*. New York: Picador USA, 1995

Carl, Dwayne. *Out of My Second Closet: Memoir of an AIDS Survivor*. Redondo Beach, CA: Nadine Kent Press, 2012

Cohen, Peter F. *Love and Anger: Essays on AIDS, Activism, and Politics*. Binghamton, NY: Hayworth Press, 1998

Gould, Deborah B. *Moving Politics: Emotion and ACT UP's Fight Against AIDS*. Chicago: University of Chicago Press, 2009

Halkaitis, Perry N. *The AIDS Generation: Stories of Survival and Resilience*. New York, NY: Oxford University Press, 2014

John, Elton. *Love is the Cure*. New York: Little, Brown and Company, 2012

Kramer, Larry. *Report from the Holocaust: The Story of an AIDS Activist*. New York: St. Martin's Press, 1994

Miller, Marla. *Deadly Little Secrets*. Kindle edition, 2013

Ruskin, Cindy. *The Quilt: Stories from the Names Project.* New York, NY: Pocket Books, 1988

Shilts, Randy. *And The Band Played On.* New York: St. Martin's Press, 1987

Various contributors. *AIDS@30.* Chicago, IL: Windy City Media Group, 2011

Angels in America: A Gay Fantasia on National Themes, a play by Tony Kushner

Common Threads: Stories from the Quilt, a documentary directed by Rob Epstein

Dallas Buyers Club, a film directed by Jean-Marc Vallee

How to Survive a Plague, a documentary directed by David France

Longtime Companion, a film directed by Norman Rene'

The Normal Heart, a play by Larry Kramer

Philadelphia, a film directed by Jonathan Demme

The Last One, a documentary directed by Nadine C. Licostie

United in Anger, a documentary produced by Jim Hubbard and Sarah Schulman

Acknowledgements:

First of all, to the people who inspired this book: the men and women with whom I worked, partied, went to school, and performed, who died from AIDS. It seems another lifetime now, but you're not forgotten.

My thanks to everyone I interviewed, but a special thanks to Michael Bongiorni with the NAMES Project/AIDS Memorial Quilt, Dwayne Carl from AIDS Project L.A., and Doneley Meris of New York HIV Arts Network.

I'm especially grateful to Tracy Baim, publisher of Windy City Media Group, for including me in their remarkable *AIDS@30 series* in 2011 and being such a great source of information and support.

My thanks to my readers – David Beckwith, Dwayne Carl, Kathy Pooler and Fredda Wasserman – for their support and insights.

And as always, to my family for their patience.

AIDS Resources:

These are some of the organizations I've worked with and researched. If you are looking for groups focused on education, testing, treatment and advocacy, they can help:

Names Memorial Project/AIDS Quilt: www.aidsquilt.org

Elton John AIDS Foundation: www.ejaf.org

AIDS Project LA: www.apla.org

American Foundation for AIDS Research: www.amfAR.org

ACT UP New York: www.actupny.com

Centers for Disease Control: www.cdc.gov

World AIDS Day: www.worldaidsday.org

Visual AIDS: www.visualaids.org

www.AIDS.gov

www.UNAIDS.org

Other books by Victoria Noe:

Friend Grief and Anger:
When Your Friend Dies and No One Gives A Damn

Friend Grief and 9/11: The Forgotten Mourners

Friend Grief and Community: Band of Friends

Friend Grief in the Workplace:
More Than An Empty Cubicle

Friend Grief and Men: Defying Stereotypes

For more information:
www.VictoriaNoe.com

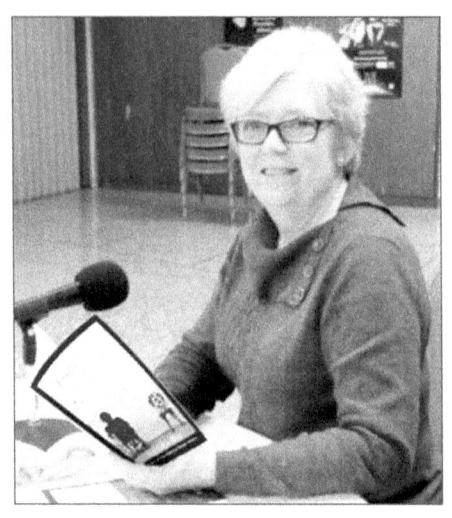

I've been a writer most of my life, but didn't admit it until 2009.

After earning a master's degree in Speech and Dramatic Art from the University of Iowa, I moved to Chicago, where I worked professionally as a stage manager, director and administrator in addition to being a founding board member of the League of Chicago Theatres. I discovered I was good at fundraising, and ventured out on my own, raising millions for arts, educational and AIDS service organizations, and later became an award-winning sales consultant of children's books. But when a concussion ended my sales career, I decided to finally keep a promise to a dying friend to write a book.

That book became a series of small books. *Friend Grief and Anger: When Your Friend Dies and No One Gives A Damn; Friend Grief and AIDS: Thirty Years of Burying Our Friends;*

Friend Grief and 9/11: The Forgotten Mourners; Friend Grief and the Military: Band of Friends (Honorable Mention, 2015 Chicago Writers Association Book of the Year Awards); *Friend Grief in the Workplace: More Than an Empty Cubicle* and *Friend Grief and Men: Defying Stereotypes.*

Next is *Fag Hags, Divas and Moms: The Legacy of Straight Women in the AIDS Community,* coming in 2017.

Among awards, my blog was named a top ten grief support website in 2012. In October, 2015, Library Journal named me their first SELF-e Ambassador. The first four e-books in the *Friend Grief* series are included in their Illinois and National collections. I've spoken at events around the country, including Book Expo America, Chicago Self-Publishing Meetup, The Muse and the Marketplace, UPublishU, Writers Digest Conference, Chicago Writers Association, public libraries and other venues.

I'm a card-carrying member of Alliance of Independent Authors (ALLi), Chicago Writers Association and ACT UP/NY (just kidding – we don't have membership cards in ACT UP).

My articles have appeared on a variety of grief and writing blogs as well as *Windy City Times, Chicago Tribune* and *Huffington Post.* My essay, "Long Term Survivor" won the 2015 Christopher Hewitt Award for Creative Nonfiction from *A&U Magazine.* In my copious spare time, I feed my reading habit by reviewing a wide variety of books on BroadwayWorld.com. A native St. Louisan, I'm a lifelong Cardinals fan and will gladly take on any comers in musical theatre trivia.

www.ingramcontent.com/pod-product-compliance
Lightning Source LLC
Chambersburg PA
CBHW072021290426
44109CB00018B/2304